GOD'S WORD IS A MEDICINE

By: Frank Baio

God's Word is a Medicine - ISBN: 9798323894864

By: Frank Baio

Unless otherwise indicated, all Scripture quotations are taken from *the King James Version* of the Holy Bible. ©1982 by Thomas Nelson, Inc. The KJV is public domain in the United States of America. Italics in the text demonstrate the author's emphasis.

Scripture quotations marked AMP are taken from *The Amplified® Bible*. Old Testament copyright©1965, 1987 by Zondervan Corporation. New Testament copyright©1958, 1987 by the Lochman Foundation. Used by permission.

Scripture quotations marked NIV are from *The New International Version®, NIV®* of the Holy Bible. Copyright ©1973, 1978 1984, 2011 by Biblica, Inc.™. Used by permission. All rights reserved worldwide.

I have used many sources, and I have attempted to cite any exact quotations and /or use material that is not under copyright. Any failure to cite a quote is simply and oversight on my part.

TABLE OF CONTENTS

~CHAPTER 1~
WHAT IS GOD'S MEDICINE?

"My son, attend to my words; consent and submit to my sayings. Let them not depart from your sight; keep them in the center of your heart. For they are life to those who find them, healing, and health to all their flesh."

Proverbs 4:20 – 22 (AMP)

The Hebrew word for "health," in verse 22, is "medicine." God's Word is medicine to all our flesh.

"...For I am the Lord who heals you," *Exodus 15:26 (AMP)* translates**, "I, the Lord am thy physician."** The medicine He prescribes is His Word.

Many make the mistake of substituting belief in healing for the actual taking of God's medicine – His Word. They say, "I believe in healing," without actually taking the medicine. What good does it do to believe in food if you do not eat? You would starve. What good does it do to believe in water if you never drink it? You would die of thirst.

God's Word is His medicine. There are several parallels between God's medicine and natural medicine.

First, God's Word is a healing agent or catalyst just as natural medicine is a healing agent or catalyst. Medicine has the ability to produce healing. God's Word contains inherently. within it the capacity, the energy, and the ability in nature to effect healing in the body.

"He sends forth His Word and heals them and rescues them from the pit of destruction."

Psalm 107:20 (AMP)

*"For they (*His Words*) are life to those that find them, healing and health to all their flesh."*

Proverbs 4:22 (AMP)

"…So shall My Word be that goes forth out of My mouth: it shall not return to Me void [without producing any effect, useless], but it shall accomplish that which I please and purpose, and it shall prosper in the thing for which I sent it.

Isaiah 55:10, 11 (AMP)

The Word, itself, contains the power to produce what it says. When God said, "Let there be light," light was. That power and authority produces healing.

"For the Word that God speaks is alive and full of power [making it active, operative, energizing, and effective]; it is sharper than any two-edged sword, penetrating to the dividing line of the breath of life (soul) and [the immortal] spirit, and of joints and marrow [of the deepest parts of our nature], exposing and sifting and analyzing and judging the very thoughts and purposes of the heart."

Hebrews 4:12 (AMP)

The key to partaking of the life and healing energy in the Word is feeding on it until it penetrates your spirit where it deposits that life and energy.

Second, medicine is not a respecter of people. It will work for anyone who takes it. It is not a matter of God willing or not willing the healing of any individual, but if the individual will receive healing by taking the medicine that produces that healing.

Third and most importantly, take the medicine according to the directions to be effective. Some medicine labels read, "Take internally," while others say, "Take externally." To rub it on your body externally when the directions say to take it internally will not work. To take it after meals when the directions say to take it before meals will reduce its effectiveness. To take it occasionally when the directions say take it three times every day will mean limited results, if any. No matter how good the medicine is, one needs to take it according to directions or it will not work. It is the same with God's medicine. You will find directions for taking God's medicine in ***Proverbs 4:20 – 22 (AMP)***

"Attend to them (God's Words) incline your ear to them, do not let them depart from before your eyes, and keep them in the midst of your heart, for they are life unto those that find them, and health to all their flesh."

NOTE: Only as God's Word gets in the midst of your heart and stays there will it produce healing in your body. Head knowledge will not do. His Word must penetrate your spirit through meditation, attending, hearing, looking, and pondering in order to produce healing for your body. Once the Word penetrates, it will surely bring health to all flesh.

*"Listen, son of mine, to what I say. Listen carefully. Keep
these thoughts ever in mind; let them penetrate deep within your
heart, for they will mean real life for you and radiant health."*

Proverbs 4:20 – 22 (LVB)

God's way of healing is spiritual. Power ministered first to your spirit, and then spread throughout your body. Take God's medicine internally.

Instead of wondering whether you have enough faith, just take the medicine! The medicine will work if you get it inside you.

Fourth, remember that it takes time for medicine to work. Most people give natural medicine <u>time</u>, <u>patience,</u> and <u>money</u> to work. They take the prescription back for refills. They are diligent about it. They do not take one dose and expect a miracle. Keep taking God's medicine. Give time for it to work.

TAKE YOUR MEDICINE!

~CHAPTER 2~
SELAH

Selah is an unusual word in scripture. As a former pastor and teacher, I have found that most people who read the Bible do not understand this word. Strong's Exhaustive Concordance says, "*Selah* means to pause."

A better definition would be to ponder, consider, wait, meditate, or think on these things.

In our fast-food mentality lives, we do things in a hurry: eating, drinking, going to work, hurrying here and there. At the end of our day, we collapse from exhaustion. It seems that man does not have any time for God.

However, God is still saying, *"Selah."* He still is asking "will you spend some time with Me. You spend so much time on unimportant things."

"This Book of the Law shall not depart out of your mouth; but you shall mediate (Selah) on it day and night, that you may observe and do according to all that is written in it. For then you all shall make your way <u>prosperous,</u> and then you shall deal wisely and have good <u>success.</u> Have I not commanded you? Be strong, vigorous, and very courageous. Be not afraid, neither be dismayed, for the Lord your God is with you wherever you go." Joshua 1:8, 9 (AMP)

Joshua learned this lesson, for we read in the Scriptures the results. As one of God' great generals, Joshua subdued 31 kings. He led the children of Israel into the land of promise.

The Bible tells us that when we are in right standing with God (righteous), then "favor goes before us" as a shield.

At the age of 110, Joshua declared boldly, *"…but as for me and my house, we will serve the Lord." Joshua 24:15b and Joshua 24:29 (AMP)*

"And it shall come to pass in that day, that his burden shall be taken away from off thy shoulder, and his yoke from off thy neck, and the yoke shall be destroyed because of the anointing."

Isaiah 10:27 (KJV)

The anointing is the burden lifting, yoke destroying, life-changing power of God. When the anointing is present, sickness <u>must</u> go, and disease <u>must</u> flee. If you feel the weight of sickness, disease, fear, depression or whatever it is that has stolen your peace, begin to meditate *(Selah)* on God's Word. Let this medicine get into your system, into your spirit and into your mind.

~CHAPTER 3~
SOTERIA (SOZO)

Many Christians today have not truly understood their salvation. If you ask them what benefit is there in being a Christian, they would not be able to tell you. Is it any wonder that so many Christians go through life defeated? Seemingly, they never walk in victory. How can this be? Well, friend, the answer is simple: They have never read the Bible with their spiritual eyes opened.

"Study to shew thyself approved unto God, a workman that needeth not to be ashamed, <u>rightly dividing</u> the word of truth."

2 Timothy 2:15 (KJV)

Let us look at our Salvation. The most important element about our Salvation is that Jesus Christ *(The Son of the Living God)* died on an old, rugged cross for our sins. In addition to dying for our sins, it states in Isaiah and Peter, *"…by his stripes we are/were healed."* **<u>PRAISE GOD FOR HIS PROVISION</u>**. Thus far, we have seen that Salvation means Redemption (forgiveness of our sins) and Healing (body, soul, and spirit).

A further study of the word Soteria/sozo, (sozo – the root word for Soteria), shows us that we have Deliverance, Provision, Prosperity, Protection, Healing, Health, Safety and Redemption. (Strong's Exhaustive Concordance)

God is so great! He has not only provided Redemption and Deliverance for us, but also Healing, Health, Provision, Prosperity, Protection and Safety. Just think about this for a moment. Our God knows all about us. We have disappointed Him so many times and yet *John 3:16 – 17 (KJV)* tells us:

"For God so loved the world that he gave his only begotten Son, that whosoever believeth in him should not perish, but have everlasting life. For God sent not his Son into the world to condemn the world, but that the world through him might be saved (Forgiven, Delivered, Protected, Provided for, be in Divine Health, Healing, Safety and Prosperous).

Because Jesus Christ, the Son of God died for us, all this is possible. Jesus paid the price for us. Yes, He paid the price for our deliverance, for our protection, for our provision, for our healing, for our health, for our safety, prosperity and for our forgiveness. Because of the finished work Jesus accomplished for us, we can now approach God as His sons and daughters. When we approach Him with this understanding, He says,

"Ask, and it shall be given to you.

seek, and ye shall find, knock,

and it shall be opened unto you."

Matthew 7:7 (KJV)

YES! ASK AND RECEIVE TODAY!

~CHAPTER 4~
THE DIFFERENCE BETWEEN HEALINGS AND MIRACLES

"Ye ask, and receive not, because ye ask amiss…"

James 4:3 (KJV).

Many people are confused about the difference between healing and miracles; let us examine these two.

Healings

Previously, we mentioned that **1 Peter 2:24 (KJV)** says, ***"Who his own self bare our sins in his own body on the tree, that we, being dead to sins, should live unto righteousness: by whose stripes ye were healed."***

Webster's Dictionary defines heal (healing) as "to become well or to become whole again; to restore someone to health; to restore (a diseased or damaged bone or tissue or wound) to its normal condition."

Divine Intervention

Healing comes about in three ways.

The **first** is through divine intervention. In short, God does it over a period of time. Healings are progressional. That means that this type of healing will take time. In the scripture, we see that ten people with leprosy came to Jesus for healing. Leprosy was the same as aids in our day. After Jesus prayed for them, He said, **"Go! Present yourselves to the priests, so that they will declare you clean (healed)."**

Notice: There were no visible signs of any change. After a while, one person with leprosy returned and knelt down to thank Jesus for healing him. On their way to see the priests, they realized that something happened. However, like many of us, only one returned to thank Jesus.

Medicines

The **second** way that a person is healed is with medicine. If you had a cough, you would take cough medicine. You will notice that your cough will subside gradually. If a physician prescribed your medication, he would insist that you take all the prescribed medicine, so to insure your healing.

Healing

The **third** way healing takes place is when the body takes over and begins the healing process. We have heard physicians say, "We have done all we can, we will have to wait and see how the patient responds to the treatment or medicine." People who suffer with broken bones require a healing process, after the bones have been set and put into a cast.

Miracles

Bill and Gloria Gaither wrote a song, "I Expect a Miracle." They defined a miracle as anticipating the inevitable, supernatural intervention of God.

Webster's Dictionary defines a miracle as "A supernatural event regarded as due to a divine action, i.e., Jesus of the Bible performed miracles. He turned water into wine, fed the five thousand, raised the dead, instantly caused the blind to see, the deaf to hear and people with disabilities to walk." Yes, these are miracles.

I have found that by taking God's medicine daily, I can use His Word not only for myself, but also for others. If you are a believer in Jesus, you can lay hands on the sick, they will recover, sometimes through healings and on other occasions we have seen miracles, (see chapter on modern day examples of healing. Praise is to Jesus! All glory to God.

"…Not by might, nor by power, but by my spirit, saith the Lord of hosts."

Zechariah 4:6 (KJV)

"And these signs shall follow them that believe; In my name shall they cast out devils; they shall speak with new tongues; They shall take up serpents; and if they drink any deadly thing, it shall not hurt them; they shall lay hands on the sick, and they shall recover. So then, after the Lord had spoken unto them, he was received up into heaven, and sat on the right hand of God. And they went forth, and preached everywhere, the Lord working with them, and <u>confirming the word with signs following</u>. Amen.

Mark 16:17 – 20 (KJV)

~Chapter 5~
10 Facts About Miracles That Will Build Your Faith

The word miracle is used to describe everything from healing a paralytic to finding a parking space at the mall on the day before Christmas. So, we begin the ten things we should all know about miracles with a definition.

A Miracle is the anticipated inevitable intervention of God!

it is an **extraordinary or startling observable event**; it **cannot reasonably be explained** in terms of human abilities or other known forces in the world; it is **perceived as a direct act of God**; and it is **usually understood to have symbolic or sign value** (e.g., pointing to God as redeemer and judge).

Part of the problem is that many Christians envision God as remote from the world, removed from any direct involvement in their lives daily. Yet numerous texts assert God's immediate involvement in everything from the growth of a blade of grass (Psalms 104) to the sustaining of our very lives (Acts 17; Colossians 1:17). For this reason, we must reject the definition of a miracle as a direct intervention of God into the world. The phrase "intervention into" implies that God is outside the world and only occasionally intrudes in its affairs.

1. God can work outside (or within) the natural realm to bring about a miracle.

Some define a miracle as God working in the world apart from means or an instrument, that would bring about the desired result. But God often uses instruments in performing the miraculous, as in the case of Jesus' feeding of the five thousand using multiplying one little boy's lunch.

Others define a miracle as God acting contrary to natural law. But this implies there are forces (natural laws) that operate independently of God, forces, or laws that God must violate or override to perform a miracle. But God is the author and providential Lord over all natural processes.

A more helpful definition of "miracle":

Wayne Grudem has proposed a definition that avoids the virus of deism while seeking to remain faithful to the Scriptures: "A miracle," says Grudem, "is a **less common kind of God's activity in which he arouses people's awe and wonder, and bears witness to himself.**" What is important for us to remember is that no matter how we define a miracle, **we must not think that a miracle means a typically absent God is now present.**

Rather, the God who is always and everywhere present, upholding and sustaining and directing all things to their appointed consummation, is now working in a surprising and unfamiliar way. This also helps us answer the question of whether unusual answers to prayer are miracles. I would say yes—if such answers are sufficiently unusual to arouse awe and wonder and to evoke acknowledgment of God's power and activity (e.g., **1 Kings 18:24**, 36-38; **Acts 12:5-17**; 28:8).

2. Miracles are part of the work of the Spirit.

It will help us to understand miracles by looking at **Galatians 3:1-5** where the apostle Paul clearly describes both the initial reception of the Spirit at the moment of salvation ("Let me ask you only this: Did you receive the Spirit by works of the law or by hearing with faith?" v. 2) and the on-going supply and provision of the Spirit throughout the course of the Christian life ("Does he who supplies the Spirit to you and works miracles among you do so by works of the law, or by hearing with faith?" v. 5).

3. We do not "earn" miracles by doing good.

God never gives his Spirit at any time or works miracles because we have put him in our debt by doing good things. Obedience to the law, says Paul, is not the reason why or the instrument through which God gives his Spirit to his people, whether that be at the point of their conversion or at any time during their Christian lives. In other words, Paul is ruling out any form of legalism or works-based approach to our experience of the Spirit. Twice in this paragraph, first in v. 2 and then again in v. 5, Paul rules out "works of the law" as the reason why we experience God's Spirit.

4. Faith is the ground for our experience of miracles.

Just as clearly as Paul ruled out works as the reason why we receive God's Spirit he affirms that faith is the cause, faith is the instrument, and faith is the grounds for our experience of the Spirit. Again, in both v. 2 and in v. 5 it is "by hearing with faith" that God bestows his Spirit. It is when we believe and trust God and his promises that he is pleased to pour out his Spirit, not only to save us and cause the Spirit to indwell us permanently (v. 2) but also to work miracles in our midst.

5. The faith to experience miracles comes from hearing...

The faith to which God responds by giving us his Spirit comes by "hearing." Hearing what? We "hear" the word of God when it is proclaimed or taught or read. Anytime the truth about God and the gospel of Jesus Christ is heard and believed and trusted and treasured and embraced, God responds by pouring out his Spirit.

5. ...but hearing must be followed by faith.

Merely "hearing" is not enough. We must have "faith" in what we have heard. Simply listening to a sermon is not enough. Just reading your Bible is not enough. Memorizing Scripture is wonderful, but if you do not believe what you have memorized it serves no good end. Reading theology books is wonderful, but if you never move beyond understanding to faith in what you have read, it profits you nothing. God does not reward us with the Spirit simply because we are smart or well-educated. People can know a lot about the Bible and can out-argue anyone theologically and never be the recipient of the miracle-working power of the Spirit.

In both **Galatians 3:2** and 5 Paul says that our hearing must be the sort that leads to faith. In other words, we have to "believe in" and "trust" and "treasure" what God has taught us or said to us in his Word. That is what pleases God. That is what serves as the instrument through which he pours out his Spirit.

6. God promises to supply His Spirit - continually.

Observe closely how God himself is described in **Galatians 3:5**. He is portrayed as "he who supplies the Spirit to you." This is a present tense participle. In other words, God is by his very nature and also by his choice a God who loves to give more of his Spirit to his people when they humble themselves and trust the truth of his Word. This is almost a badge of identification. God is saying, "This is who I am. This is what I do. I continually supply the Spirit to my people."

7. Miracles - and other provisions of the Spirit - happen among God's people.

Do not forget that Paul is writing to Christians! These people in Galatia have already trusted Christ for their salvation. Back in **Galatians 3:2,** Paul referred to the provision of the Spirit that God made to them when they first trusted Jesus for salvation. But now in **Galatians 3:5,** he is saying that God continues to make provision for believing men and women. I stress this point simply because this is one verse that should forever put to rest the debate about whether God continues after our conversion to supply and provide us with more and more of the Spirit. He does not call this experience in **Galatians 3:5** "Spirit baptism" or "Spirit filling." He does not use the word "anointing." But does it matter? All that matters is that God is the sort of God whose very nature and purpose it is to give more of his Spirit on an ongoing, daily basis to his people.

8. We need to have confidence in the character of God...

What specifically is it that God wants us to believe? In other words, what is the content or object of our "faith" to which God answers with the extraordinary supply and provision of his Spirit? We are not told explicitly, but I know. There are several things Paul likely has in mind.

Given the larger context and purpose of the letter to the Galatians, he surely has in mind our faith in the finality of Christ's death and resurrection and our confidence in that gracious work of God as the only hope for salvation. In other words, believing that we are justified by faith alone, through grace alone, in Christ alone is central to what we must believe. This is obvious when we read on in v. 6 of **Galatians 5** where Paul speaks of Abraham "believing" God and being justified as a result.

Paul has in mind our faith and confidence in the character of God. Do you believe God is the sort of God who loves to do wonderful things for his people? Do you believe God is the kind of God who delights to build up and restore and heal? Do you believe that God is of such a character and nature that he has compassion on his people and rejoices to do them good at all times? Believing this about God is crucial to our experience of the supernatural work of the Spirit.

8b. ...and know He can do things.

Related to the former point is our faith that God can do such things. You may think that goes without saying. Surely if you are a Christian you know and are confident that God can do miraculous things for us. But may I remind you that Jesus always responded to that sort of faith with healing and deliverance and blessing. Let me give you a couple of examples of this. In **Matthew 9:28-29** Jesus said this to two blind men: "Do you believe that I can do this?" They said to him, "Yes, Lord." Then Jesus touched their eyes saying, "According to your faith be it done to you." And they were instantly healed.

According to what "faith"? What exactly had they believed that led Jesus to heal them? It was not their belief or faith that it was his "will" to heal them. Jesus never asked them, "Do you believe that I am willing to heal you?" He merely asked if they believed he was "able" to heal them and when they said Yes, he healed them.

The leper in **Matthew 8** said to Jesus, "Lord, if you are willing, you can make me clean" (v. 2). The leper did not question Christ's ability. He trusted that completely. He did have doubts about the willingness of Jesus to do it. But Jesus did not rebuke him for such doubts, as if it were a shortcoming in his faith that might jeopardize his healing. He healed him because of his confidence that he could do it.

9. Miracles were not just the work of apostles – they happened among average Christians.

God is working miracles among and through these Galatian Christians in the absence of any apostolic influence. As far as we know, there were no apostles present in Galatia when Paul wrote this. Thus, contrary to what most cessationists say, miracles were not exclusively or even primarily the work of apostles but were typically found among ordinary, average Christians like those in first-century Galatia.

10. The word often translated as "miracles" in 1 Corinthians 12:10 is the Greek word for "powers".

In conclusion, consider how this passage relates to what Paul says in **1 Corinthians 12:10** and the spiritual gift of "miracles". The most literal translation of Paul's words in **1 Corinthians 12:10** is "workings of powers" (energemata dunameon). Although all gifts are "workings" (energemata) or "energizing" by divine power (compared to vv. 6, 11), the word is used here in conjunction with "powers" (dunamis) for a particular gift. The word often translated as "miracles" in **1 Corinthians 12:10** is actually the Greek word for powers (dunamis). Thus, we again have a double plural, "workings of powers," which probably points to a certain variety in these operations.

So, does God "work miracles" among us, or do gifted individuals "work miracles" among us? Yes! God "works miracles" among us by awakening faith in his Word, in conjunction with or as a result of which he imparts a gracious divine enabling (i.e., a charisma, a gift) so that the believer can "work miracles" among us.

Finally, what are these "workings" or "effects" or "productions" of "powers"?

"Workings," "effects," "productions," and "powers":

Whereas all the gifts mentioned in 1 Corinthians 12:8-10 are certainly miraculous, the gift of miracles must primarily encompass other supernatural phenomena as well. Simply put, whereas all healings and prophetic words are displays of power, not all displays of power result in healing or prophetic words.

Several possible manifestations of divine power may be included in what Paul means by "workings of powers" or "miracles." Consider the following: see Acts 9:40 where Peter raised Tabitha/Dorcas from the dead (although even this is a healing in the strictest sense of the term). Or consider Acts 13:8-11 where Paul induced blindness on Elymas. One might also include here Peter's word of disciplinary judgment that resulted in the immediate death of Ananias and Sapphira (Acts 5:1-11). Perhaps nature miracles would be included here, such as turning water to wine, stilling the storm on the Sea of Galilee, reproducing food, and causing the rain to cease (or commence), as with Elijah. We might also include supernatural deliverances (exorcisms) are in view as well.

~Chapter 6~
Healing Is the Children's (Believers) Bread!

"22 And behold, a woman who was a Canaanite from that district came out and, with a [loud, troublesomely urgent] cry, begged, Have mercy on me, O Lord, Son of David! My daughter is miserably and distressingly and cruelly possessed by a demon!

23 But He did not answer her a word. And His disciples came and implored Him, saying; Send her away, for she is crying out after us.

24 He answered, "I was sent only to the lost sheep of the house of Israel."

26 And He answered, "It is not right (proper, becoming, or fair) to take the children's bread and throw it to the little dogs."

27 She said, "Yes, Lord, yet even the little pups (little whelps) eat the crumbs that fall from their [young] masters' table

28 Then Jesus answered her, "O woman, great is your faith! Be it done for you as you wish." And her daughter was cured from that moment."

Matthew 15:22-28 (AMP)

<u>Jesus is saying here that healing is a staple of life. As Bread is a staple of life so is healing.</u>

Bread the Staple (Staff) of Life

As a principle food for the human body bread, has played a major role in keeping humans alive. Bread is considered a staple food—i.e., a basic dietary item. A person can survive a long time on only bread and water. Bread is such a basic food item that it becomes synonymous for food in general.

Staff of life - *A staple or necessary food, especially bread. For example, Rice is the staff of life for a majority of the earth's people. This expression, which uses staff in the sense of "a support," was first recorded in 1638.*

"3 And when the tempter came to him, he said, "If thou be the Son of God, command that these stones be made BREAD."

4 But he answered and said, "It is written, Man shall not live by bread alone, but by EVERY WORD that proceedeth out of the mouth of God.""

Matt 4:3-4 (KJV)

EAT the WORD of HEALING like bread.

"16 THY WORDS were found, and I did EAT THEM; and THY WORD was unto me the joy and rejoicing of mine heart: for I am called by thy name, O LORD God of hosts."

Jeremiah 15:16 (KJV)

EAT (take) the WORD of HEALING like medicine

If you are in need for healing or a miracle, you too can act like this gentile woman. No one could doubt that it was a bold move.

After all, she was a "gentile," a woman outside the covenant of God. They were referred to, by the Jews of her day, as mere "dogs." But she was a typical mother who loved her daughter with an undying love. She had watched the torment day after day, month after month, and a person can only endure just so much. She had been to all of the doctors. She had even sought the advice of her religious leaders and the advice of her friends. Nothing. They all had nothing to offer. She was desperate and something had to be done!

She had heard of a prophet that was in the region, one that some were calling the Messiah. It was well known that the Jews were expecting the coming Messiah which was spoken of in the ancient writings. Could this really be Him? Surely the miracles she had heard about substantiated such a claim. Wherever He went there seemed to be hope. Life seemed to spring forth from Him as impossible situations were turned around. Yes, she had heard the stories and of His great compassion, and as if a dream had come true, here He was in her own hometown, and she believed.

With the boldness of a lion, she cast aside the fact that she was a gentile and approached Jesus for the healing of her daughter. Jesus paused and did not answer right away. The disciples came and asked if they should send her away, as she was such a bother and making such a scene.

Then Jesus stopped, turned, and looked her square in the eyes and said, "I was not sent except to the lost sheep of the house of Israel." Momentarily stunned by His answer, she could not deny that she knew down deep within herself that there was no other hope. She knew that He was the author of life, that He had all authority, and she humbled herself and worshiped Him and simply said; "Help me!"

Jesus answered her with a very profound phrase; "It is not good to take the children's bread and throw it to the little dogs." She understood clearly her place of unrighteousness, and yet having heard of the mercy of God, she replies meekly by saying; "Yes, Lord, yet even the little dogs eat the crumbs which fall from their masters table."

What would you do if Jesus had been this rude to you, as it seems that He was with this woman? Would you have gotten angry? Would you have been insulted?

Yet, this woman demonstrated humility by swallowing her pride. Her need was greater than her pride. This was when true faith arose in her. She knew that all Jesus had to do was to say the word and her daughter would be delivered. Her declaration opened the door for the bread (healing) to be released. The faith she demonstrated was not based on expectation, but rather it was based on knowing and knowing (the assurance) that her miracle was already accomplished.

Jesus marveled at the woman's reply and her unwillingness to let go of the truth, stating that she had great faith. Then with that look of compassionate assurance, He said to her; "Let it be as you desire." And her daughter was healed!

Did you catch what Jesus said about healing? He referred to healing as the "children's bread." In other words, healing is the rightful, normal, expected sustenance of the children of God - it is their inheritance! I have found that many Christians are really not sure if healing belongs to them through the redemptive plan of salvation. Unfortunately, there is often an uncertainty about this issue. Know this - uncertainty is always an open door for the enemy to sow confusion, and a breeding ground for fear, doubt, and unbelief. As believers, we need to have our feet planted upon solid ground, knowing with all certainty that which belongs to us, so that we can apply the Word of God in any given situation and therefore receive the promised benefit. Where do you stand? Are you a child of God? Have you asked Jesus to come into your heart? If you answered, yes, then the right of healing is yours today, now, right at this moment - just as it was then, it is still the children's bread today.

True Bible faith can only act where the will of God is known. That is why we have the Bible today; it is His will in written form. This woman had a revelation or an understanding that Jesus was the Messiah, that He was not only *able* to heal, but that He was *willing* to do so. Based on that understanding, she was not going to let Jesus pass her by. She had boldness as a result of her faith that was based upon knowledge, and she acted on it. In a sense she was saying - ***I know the truth and I will not be denied!***

In Matthew 6, Jesus introduces what is commonly known as the Lord's Prayer. This should more accurately be referred to as the disciple's prayer. (This was to teach the disciples how to pray). In this prayer (verse 11) Jesus says when praying to the Father, "Give us this day our daily bread". For years we had been taught that we need to pray for our daily provision. However, now we know that bread is not only our daily provision but our healing (health) as well

"I am the bread of life." John 6:48

'I am the living bread which came down from heaven. If anyone eats of this bread, he will live forever; and the bread that I shall give is My flesh, which I shall give for the life of the world." John 6:51

Eat The Word. The Word is your medicine. A scripture a day keeps the doctor away!

~CHAPTER 7~
WHAT THE BIBLE SAYS ABOUT HEALING

Many people who needed healing went looking for Jesus. They came from everywhere so that Jesus would touch them. One of the greatest qualities that Jesus demonstrated was His compassion for hurting people. His compassion moved Him to action. The Word of God says of Jesus, "He is the same yesterday, today and forever." Jesus is still demonstrating that compassion today, as He did in New Testament days. **YES, HE WANTS TO HEAL YOU TODAY. WILL YOU TRUST AND BELIEVE THAT HE WILL?**

"Who his own self bare our sins in his own body on the tree, that we, being dead to sins, should live unto righteousness: by whose stripes ye were healed."

1 Peter 2:24 (KJV)

"…by his wounds you have been healed."

(AMP)

"If you will diligently hearken to the voice of the Lord your God and will listen to what is right in His sight and will listen to and obey His commandments and keep all His statutes, I will put none of the diseases upon you which I brought upon the Egyptians, for I am the Lord Who (continually) heals you."

Exodus 15:26 (AMP)

God is speaking to you now, saying, "I am the Lord that healeth thee." He is watching over His Word to perform it. He is the Lord that heals you. He is healing you now. His Word contains the ability to produce what it says. His Word is full of healing power. Say aloud: I receive the healing that is in His Word now!

Healing is inherent in God's nature. God is in us. Our bodies are the temples of God. Our bodies are the temples of the Lord that heals us. God is dwelling inside us, healing us now.

Father, I thank You because You are my healer. You are healing me now.

"And ye shall serve the Lord your God, and He shall bless thy bread, and thy water; and I will take sickness away from the midst of thee."

Exodus 23:25 (KJV)

``You shall serve the Lord your God only; then I will bless you with food and with water, and I will take away sickness from among you."

Exodus 23:23 (LVB)

("I Will" is the strongest assertion made in the English language.)

"Why art thou cast down, O my soul? And why art thou disquieted within me? Hope thou in God, for I shall yet praise Him, who is the health of my countenance, and my God."

Psalms 42:11 (KJV)

Father, I praise You because You are the health of my countenance.

"He that dwelleth in the secret place of the most High shall abide under the shadow of the Almighty. I will say of the Lord, He is my refuge and my fortress: my God; in Him will I trust. Surely, He shall deliver thee from the snare of the fowler, and from the noisome pestilence. He shall cover thee with His feathers and under His wings shalt thou trust; His truth shall be thy shield and buckler. Thou shalt not be afraid for the terror by night; nor for the arrow that fleeth by day; Nor for the pestilence that walketh in darkness; nor for the destruction that wasted at noonday."

Psalm 91:1 – 6 (KJV)

"He that dwells in the secret place of the Most High shall remain stable and fixed under the shadow of the Almighty (Whose power no foe can withstand).

Psalms 91:1 (AMP)

"We live within the shadow of the Almighty, sheltered by the God who is above all gods. This I declare that He alone is my refuge, my place of safety; He is my God, and I am trusting Him. For He rescues you from every trap and protects you from the fatal plague. He will shield you with His wings! They will shelter you. His faithful promises are your armor. Now you do not need to be afraid of the dark anymore, nor fear the dangers of the day; nor dread the plagues of darkness, nor disasters in the morning.

Psalm 91:1 – 6 (LVB)

"Bless the Lord, O my soul, and forget not all His benefits: Who forgives all thine iniquities, who healeth all thy diseases."

Psalm 103:2, 3 (KJV)

"He sent His Word, and healed them, and delivered them from their destructions."

Psalm 107:20 (KJV)

"He sent His Word to heal them and preserve their life."

Psalm 107:20 (Moffat)

"…and there is healing in His wings."

Malachi 4:2 (KJV)

We see in these Scriptures that we can say we are not afraid of disease. I am not afraid of sickness. I am abiding in the shadow of **Jehova-Rapha** (I am the God that healeth thee). No plague shall come nigh my dwelling or my body. I resist sickness and disease. Sickness (name it), you cannot come nigh my dwelling.

"…and with His stripes we are healed."

Isaiah 53:6 (KJV)

"…by whose stripes' ye were healed."

1 Peter 2:24 (KJV)

In these Scriptures respectively, we read the words **are** and **were**. Both Isaiah and Peter were looking at healing from two sides of Calvary's cross.

Isaiah was looking toward the cross to what it would provide.

Peter, on the other hand, is looking at what the cross has already (accomplished) provided.

~CHAPTER 8~
HOW TO RECEIVE YOUR HEALING

Over the year, I have found that people will try many different means to get their healing before they resort to God. It is because they operate in the natural world. The Scriptures state that the natural man (mind) cannot comprehend the spiritual. Therefore, hurting people try different things to get their healing. Oh, how this must grieve the heart of God. What can we do to get our healing?

Dale Carnegie was quoted as saying, "What man can conceive in his mind and believe in his heart, man can (will) achieve." Let us see if this principal really works in spiritual matters, more specifically, our **healing.**

Necessity Demands Action

"And a certain woman, which had an issue of blood twelve years,

And had suffered many things of many physicians, and had spent all that she had, and was nothing bettered, but rather grew worse,

When she had heard of Jesus, came in the press behind, and touched his garment.

For she said, If I may touch but His clothes, I shall be whole.

And straightway the fountain of her blood was dried up; and she felt in her body that she was healed of that plague.

And Jesus, immediately knowing in Himself that virtue had gone out of Him, turned Him about in the press, and said, <u>Who touched my clothes?</u>

And His disciples said unto Him, Thou seest the multitude thronging Thee, and sayest Thou, Who touched me?

And He looked round about to see her that had done this thing.

But the woman fearing and trembling, knowing what was done in her, came and fell down before Him, and told Him all the truth. And He said unto her, Daughter, thy faith hath made the whole; go in peace and be whole of thy plague."

Mark 5:25 – 34 (KJV)

This Biblical account certainly fits Dale Carnegie's quote "what man can conceive and believe he can achieve." This unnamed woman definitely had a major need that required action. In order to receive her healing, she took several steps.

First, she <u>conceived</u> in her mind. She thought, "If I may touch his clothes," a glimmer of hope, is it possible?

Second, "I shall be whole!" She <u>believed it</u>. This was not a question or a half-hearted statement. This woman was not going to stop until she received her healing. She knew that she knew that she would receive her healing. There was no doubt in her mind.

Third, she took action. She <u>achieved</u>. The Scriptures tell us that she came in the press behind and touched him.

This woman is a marvelous example of how to receive healing. From the very beginning, we see that her condition was serious. She saw numerous physicians with no success. She exhausted all her savings. Her hemorrhaging had been going on for twelve long years, and what little hope she had left was slipping away.

One day, she heard some people talking about a special man named Jesus. Is it possible that what she was hearing is true? The blind got their sight. The lame walked. The dead came back to life. Is it possible that this Jesus could do for her what no other physician had been able to do? The day came that Jesus was in town. She was ready. She was going to get her healing and nothing was going to stop her.

She got herself ready and went as fast as her feet would take her in her condition. All at once, she came to a sudden stop. What is this? She had not counted on the crowd. What will she do? That is when she must have said within herself, if she could touch His garment, she knew she would be whole. She knew that necessity demanded action. She began to push her way through the crowd. She got closer and closer, just a little closer – there. In order to touch the hem of His garment, this sickly woman got down on her knees, humbled herself and touched his garment. The moment she touched the hem of His garment, something happened. It felt like a bolt of lightning and heat inside of her. It happened! She knew it.

When the woman touched Jesus, He knew that something special had just happened. He asked his disciples who touched Him. The disciples answered Jesus You must be kidding. Look around You. Do You not see the crowd? You want us to tell You who touched You.

Jesus said, "I felt virtue depart from me." What Jesus meant was that He felt anointing, healing power, flow from Him. Even though there were many people grabbing for Him, only one person was able to draw healing from Him in that instant.

This happened because of her faith. Jesus then turned to the woman and looked at her. The Scriptures tell us that the woman, with fear and trembling, came and fell down before Him and told Him the truth. Jesus said to her, "Daughter, be of good comfort; thy faith hath made thee whole."

Can you picture the celebration that there must have been in her home that night?

Dear friend, no matter how hopeless or impossible your situation may be, Jesus, our Great Physician, is still healing today.

~CHAPTER 9~
EXAMPLES OF MODERN DAY MIRACULOUS HEALINGS

In 1994, I ministered in a church in Western Pennsylvania. There was a very special presence of God in that service. I knew that God was going to do a supernatural work that day. The Pastor of the church asked to have an anointing service. For those that are unfamiliar with this type of service, I will explain. An invitation to come forward is given to the congregation (at the end of the preaching or when the Holy Spirit leads) by the speaker or the Pastor. The speaker or the Pastor dips his or her finger into the anointing oil and applies it on the congregant's forehead. This is symbolic of the Holy Spirit.

"Is any sick among you? let him call for the elders of the church; and let them pray over him, anointing him with oil in the name of the Lord: And the prayer of faith shall save the sick, and the Lord shall raise him up; and if he have committed sins, they shall have forgiven him."

James 5:14 – 15 (KJV)

The service seemed impregnated with an electrical current that you could not see, but certainly feel.

"...Not by might, nor by power, but by my spirit, saith the Lord of hosts."

Zechariah 4:6 (KJV)

All of the ingredients were there.

The praise was very powerful. The word of God says, ***"That He inhabits the praise of His people."*** As the praises went up, the power of God came down.

Then as the preaching of the Word came forth, faith began to rise. The Word says, ***"So then faith cometh by hearing, and hearing by the Word of God."*** Praise God! As the intensity builds, you know that you know that God is about to do a powerful work among His people.

When I finished preaching the Word, I gave the invitation. Almost every member of that church came forward. The Bible says, ***"Blessed are they which do hunger and thirst after righteousness: for they shall be filled."*** These people were ready to receive from God.

And these signs shall follow them that believe…they shall lay hands on the sick, and they shall recover."

Mark 16:17, 18 (KJV)

In obedience to God's Word, we began laying hands on the sick (or oppressed) and anointing them with oil. The results were immediate. The power of God seemed to sweep through the church that day. People received healing, deliverance, and the Baptism in the Holy Spirit. However, the most memorable was a certain woman. As I approached her; I asked, "What is it that you want to be prayed for? Her answer was, "I am going to the hospital for exploratory surgery. Please pray that God gives me the strength to go through it."

The Holy Spirit spoke to my mind in that instant. This is what He told me to do: "Ask her, do you believe that God can heal you? Do you believe that God wants to heal you, very much?" Her answer did not surprise me when she said, "No, I don't know, I just don't know!" I quoted Scriptures to her until I felt the release from the Holy Spirit. Then I prayed in the Spirit.

Since I did not know what her problem was, I had my wife and another woman place their hands on this woman's abdomen. I then placed my hand on their hands. As I did, I felt a current go through my arm and enter the woman. When the anointing went into her, it also entered the Pastor (who was standing behind her) who jumped backward, due to the intense anointing. We all knew that God did something for this woman, but we would not find out until later that day.

After the service, the church had a time of refreshments. As I was speaking with several of the church members, the Pastor's wife came to me and told me to go with her, someone wanted to speak with me. I followed her into the foyer and the woman for whom we prayed greeted me. This is her testimony to the Glory of God.

The reason for the exploratory surgery was that I have not had a menstrual discharge in four months. The doctors have decided to operate tomorrow morning, but PRAISE BE TO GOD when you laid your hand on me, a fire and warmth went through my body. Immediately, the flow begin and that is why I needed to go home and change. After I changed the Lord said "go and tell the man of God. what I have done for you." So here I am praising the Lord and giving Him all the glory.

PRAISE GOD! PRAISE GOD! PRAISE GOD!

RE-CREATIVE MIRACLES

I have concluded not only can God heal, but He also performs re-creative miracles. Such is the story of Sister Ann, a member of a church where I served as Associate Pastor.

At the conclusion of our weekly Thursday Morning Healing Service, I invited those who needed prayer to come forward. Sister Ann was one of those who came forward. I asked her what the need was. She said she would like to stand in proxy for her daughter who needed healing. We came into agreement.

"Again, I say unto you, "That if two of you shall agree on earth as touching anything that they shall ask, it shall be done for them of My Father which is in heaven." Matthew 18:19 (KJV)

I anointed her with oil by placing my hands over her ears. As I touched her, she reached for her ears and covered them with her hands. I just stood there not understanding what happened. Later, she testified to what took place.

When Sister Ann came forward for prayer, she was seeking prayer for her daughter, but God does far more than we can ever think or ask. She was in her 80's and had to wear hearing aids. Just prior to that service, the doctor fitted both ears for hearing aids. That Thursday morning, God healed her ears (recreated). To confirm her healing, Ann went back to her audiologist to be re-examined. The doctor ran the tests several times. When he returned, he was shaking his head saying he did not understand. He just did not understand. Ann's hearing had improved considerably, and she did not have to wear hearing aids anymore. Ann brought her test results to church to show us.

PRAISE GOD! PRAISE GOD!

HEART PROBLEMS

During a Good Friday service, God truly visited his people. The location was at a Holiday Inn in Western Pennsylvania. The conference room was full to capacity. I was one of the speakers. The Hostess was Pastor Averill Vareen. She was the Pastor of a church in Beaver Falls, Pennsylvania. Pastor Vareen invited Pastors from all denominations and multi-racial backgrounds. The common reason for our gathering was to remember what Jesus Christ accomplished on the cross.

The agenda was simple. Each invited Pastor was to speak for five minutes. Can you imagine that? Have you ever heard of a preacher speaking for only five minutes? When God is in control, all things are possible.

The service began with much prayer. Then, we sang praises and worshipped. You felt the presence of God in that room. As the worship intensified, there seemed to be a mist covering the room. The best way to describe it is this: Have you ever been in a room where there were heavy smokers? In that environment, the smoke rises to the ceiling. This smoke gave the same appearance with two major differences. The first difference being that the smoke was not foul or stale. The second was that the smoke was not rising but descending on the people. This truly was the descending Glory of God.

This presence was so powerful that people began to take their shoes off. This truly was Holy Ground. Rather than interrupting this move of the Holy Spirit, Pastor Vareen invited those that needed a healing from God to come forward for prayer. She called her son and me to assist her in praying for the sick. Many with back, neck or abdominal problems received instant healing.

Then, Pastor Vareen asked if I had heard from God? I said that I had. This is what God had given me. "Several here are suffering with heart problems. If they came, the anointing would set them free, and healing would be immediate."

NOTE: Do this with care. You do not turn on the gifts of the Spirit whenever you want to. In Corinthians, we see that the Holy Spirit will minister through whom He will, so that God would receive the glory.

Several came forward for pray. The power of god overwhelmed them. After this response, surely, God was through, but He was not. I did not feel the release from God to go on. Then I said this, "God is yet not through. There is one more person who did not come forward. You know who you are. God said that He is still waiting for you. At that moment, a woman raced forward and said that she was the one. Please pray for her. This is what she had to say.

Last night I had to call the paramedics to my home due to terrible chest pains. They said that I had all of the symptoms of a heart attack. They wanted to take me to the hospital, but I would not let them because I want to trust in my God. The reason I did not come forward sooner was that I did not have the strength. God just gave me the strength, so here I am. As soon as we prayed for her, all of her chest pains disappeared. They just stopped. PRAISE GOD!

LUMPS DISAPPEAR

We witnessed many healing and miracles in Pennsylvania, Florida, and Haiti.

One of the most memorable miracles that we witnessed took place in Florida. After a dedicatory service, I gave an invitation for those that needed prayer. A woman came forward and requested prayer. She had lumps in her breast. She said that she would have to go to a doctor. However, she believed that God was greater than the problem. I had several women place their hands on her.

We praised God for her healing (even before she received it). We felt the power of God and knew that God was ready to demonstrate His presence with His power in that church. As I laid my hand on her forehead, heat went through her body and the lumps disappeared. PRAISE GOD!

The anointing was so strong that it took two men to carry her to her car. (Her husband drove). One of the family members told us that this anointing was on for her for three days. GLORY TO GOD! PRAISE GOD! PRAISE GOD!

TUMOR VANISHES

Several years ago, we saw an incurable tumor vanish before our very eyes. It all began with friends of ours who were foster parents. They asked if we would take care of Brock and his brother, Roy, while they went on vacation. Since we already had approval from Human Resource Services (HRS), we knew all was in order.

Brock's problems were numerous: Cerebral Palsy, a massive tumor at the base of his spine paralyzed him from the waist down, and several other disorders. For a child who was almost four years old, he had a remarkable temperament. It was heartbreaking to see him drag himself across the floor while playing with the other children, just to keep up with them.

The foster parents told us that Brock was going to the Shiners' Hospital for Children in Lakeland, Florida when they returned from their vacation. The procedure in consideration for Brock was to place steel rods alongside his leg bones. The reason for this was that his upper body had grown, whereas his lower body and legs had not. The concern was that if Brock were to become over-energetic and attempt to stand, his legs would not sustain his weight. Therefore, his bones might shatter, and the splintered bones could penetrate his abdomen and cause his death.

That Sunday morning, we took Brock and Roy to church. When the Pastor gave the invitation for prayer, I went forward with Brock in my arms. Due to his size and the shape of his body, his posterior fit in the palm of my hand. You could feel the mass (tumor). Something happened that I will never forget. As the Pastor prayed and anointed Brock with oil, the mass began to shrivel up. By the time we got home, the tumor was completely gone.

Here is the amazing part. When the foster parents took Brock to the hospital for his preoperative screening (x-rays, etc.), the doctors were amazed. They could not find the tumor. The two-day screening turned into four days. The doctors asked the foster parents if they had switched children on them. Why did they ask that? What was there before was not there now. Praise God!

We have witnessed many other miracles over the years. However, we have also seen individuals who have not received a miracle or healing. In another chapter, I will discuss hindrances to healing.

~ CHAPTER 10 ~
WAYS GOD USES TO HEAL

The Laying On Of Hands

"And these signs shall follow them that believe; In my name shall they cast out devils; they shall speak with new tongues; They shall take up serpents; and if they drink any deadly thing, it shall not hurt them; they shall lay hands on the sick, and they shall recover." Mark 16:17, 18

In the Gospel of Mark, we read that Jesus gave the disciples His authority and power to preach the gospel to every creature, to heal the sick, and to raise the dead. This is the Great Commission. He did this so that they could minister in His absence. In other passages of Scripture, we find that believers laid hands on the sick and the sick recovered (healed).

We witnessed this laying of hands on the sick during a recent trip to Haiti. I was the guest speaker at a crusade held in this poverty-stricken country. After the first evening service, compelled by the Holy Spirit, I called people forward for a healing service. I was amazed at the response. Over 2,500 people came for prayer. One of our team members said it best, "It was like a sea of humanity. It was reminiscent of the crowds that must have followed Jesus. The people's needs were so great that necessity demanded action. These people wanted God to meet their needs.

We ministered to as many as we could that night. The next night, there were more people than the first night. I broke down and cried aloud to God and said, "This is too great for one person to accomplish alone." Then the Lord spoke to my heart and mind and said these simple words, "TEACH THEM."

The next day, I assembled approximately 60 local Pastors. I told them what God had shown me. There was such excitement. The text to teach these Pastors was Mark 16:17 – 18. After approximately six hours, these men were ready for that evening's service. That night was a night not soon to be forgotten.

When we arrived at the stadium, I noticed people lying on the infield (this was a soccer stadium). I asked what was happening. They told me that these were the prayer warriors interceding for the service. The praise and worship were powerful. You knew that God was about to do great work.

"Then he answered and spake unto me, saying, This is the Word of the Lord unto Zerubbabel, saying, Not by might, nor by power, but by My spirit, saith the Lord of hosts." Zechariah 4:6 (KJV)

That night a local Pastor spoke on my behalf to give my voice a rest. They asked me to give the altar call for salvation. As in previous nights, many came forward to accept Jesus as their personal Savior. If the service were to end then, it would have been worth it. However, God had more in store for us.

I instructed the Pastors to form a semicircle in front of the platform. Then, I gave the invitation to the people to come forward, but this time the Pastors laid hands on them for healing. There were hundreds upon hundreds of healing and miracles done in the name of Jesus, by the power of the Holy Spirit and by the Blood of the Lamb.

The following day was our last day in Haiti. The schedule was to conduct the Pastor's Workshop and speak in the evening service. At our workshop, I asked the Pastors to describe the events of the previous nights. One right after another, they testified of miracles and healings that God performed. At the end of our final workshop, we anointed each Pastor for the task that lay before him.

The Best Was Yet to Come

When we arrived at the stadium that evening, we knew that there was a war going on all around us, not with conventional weapons, but in the spirit and we knew it. The devil did not want this service to go.

"…IF GOD BE FOR US, WHO CAN BE AGAINST US?"

As the praise team got up to sing, we heard voodoo drums in the background. We sang with greater intensity. We preached the word, yet the battle raged on. A storm rolled in off the coast just as we gave the altar call. The threat of the storm did not stop people from responding to Jesus and accepting Him into their hearts.

Then the altar call for those needing healing was given. As the night prior, the Pastors took their place and waited for the people with a passion. Just then, it began to rain. It was a torrential outpouring. Within 20 minutes, the infield was flooded with at least two feet of water. There was lightning and thunder all around. I am convinced that the devil was throwing his best punch at us. However, God has the last word in all matters. The devil thought that he had won, but the Pastors stood their ground. As the water was rising in the infield, these anointed men and women continued to minister. By the time we left, many wheelchairs, that at one time carried the sick and the paralytic, were left behind, empty. These empty wheelchairs are a testimony of God's power.

The blind had their sight restored and the deaf heard. A four-year-old child, who was crippled from birth, was carried in her father's arms. As we prayed for her, we heard the child's bones snapping and popping into place. Her father carried her in, but now she pulled on her father's finger and ran out of the stadium. Truly, this was a work from God Almighty.

The unforgettable sight that will remain with me is the 60-plus Pastors, waist deep in water, with lightning and thunder roaring all around, laying hands on the sick, and they did recover.

Prayer Cloths

"So that from his body were brought unto the sick, handkerchiefs or aprons, and the diseases departed from them, and the evil spirits went out of them." Acts 19:12 (KJV)

There are times when necessity requires action. In this verse, we have an account where the people realized that Paul, the Apostle, could not be everywhere at the same time. The people brought aprons and handkerchiefs so that he could anoint them and when these items touched the bodies of the sick, they received their healing. We also see that even the evil spirits went out of them.

"And it shall come to pass in that day, that his burden shall be taken away from off thy shoulder, and his yoke from off thy neck, and the yoke shall be destroyed because of the anointing." Isaiah 10:27 (KJV)

In the book of Isaiah, we see a very important principle. The anointing destroys the yoke. In the book of Acts, we saw that the people brought aprons and handkerchiefs to Paul so that he could lay his hands on these items. Paul learned that the anointing is transferable. When the people place these anointed items on the bodies of the sick, the sick recovered. People need a point of contact to release their faith.

Several years ago, I attended a church that believed in using prayer clothes. They were a very effective method of ministry.

One Sunday, a woman came and requested a prayer cloth for her brother-in-law. He had had a stroke the night before. The doctors said that he would not be able to work or drive his car again. We prayed, anointing the cloth. She mailed the cloth to her brother-in-law, who lived in Virginia. Within six months, the man was speaking clearly, working, and driving his car without any problems. The doctors gave him a clean bill of health.

On another occasion, a prayer request came for a newborn child with a spinal disorder. The child had a hole at the tip of her spine. We mailed a prayer cloth to her at the hospital in Ohio. Within two or three months, the child was rolling in her crib. That was a miracle because the doctors told the family that she would be a vegetable.

PRAISE GOD! PRAISE GOD!

Anointing With Oil

"And the prayer of faith shall save the sick, and the Lord shall raise him up; and if he has committed sins, they shall be forgiven him." James 5:15 (KJV)

In the letter of James, we see that there are times when we have prayed for ourselves, or others have prayed for us, and nothing has happened. This provision is solely for the church. In this provision, a believer in a local assembly is to call for the Elder of that assembly. The Elder anoints the sick person with oil. The oil is symbolic of the Holy Spirit. In James 5:14 – 15, the Apostle, James, is making several important points:

1.   The sick person must take the first step.

2.   The Elder's prayer of faith will heal the sick.

3.   If there is any sin, they shall be forgiven him.

Many Christians get upset with their Pastors when they miss church, and the Pastor does not contact them. They get hurt. They are offended. They begin to pout. They act like children.

James is telling the Church that you are to call the Elders when you are sick. If the Pastor is the only Elder, then it is your responsibility to call him so that he can pray for you.

Praise That Heals

"But Thou art Holy, O Thou that inhabitest the praises of Israel." Psalm 22:3 (KJV)

"For where two or three are gathered together in My name, there am I in the midst of them." Matthew 18:20 (KJV)

Our praise creates the environment in which God operates. In both of these passages, God set up another method for us to receive our healing. I know this firsthand; you see it happened to me.

For 29 years, I suffered from bronchitis. I went to the Veterans Hospital at Bay Pines in St. Petersburg, Florida. When the doctor examined me, he said that I had to have an X-ray taken. Then, I needed to have a blood test. Before I left the hospital, the results came back on the blood test and X-ray. The blood test was negative. Praise God! However, the X-ray showed a mass on one of the lungs. They scheduled a CAT SCAN to be on the safe side.

Two weeks later, I went for the CAT SCAN, and then the wait. The CAT SCAN confirmed the mass and nothing more. The doctor said that he wanted me to return within two weeks for possible treatment. Even though he did not mention the "C" word, (cancer), that is what the doctor was leaning toward. God's Word says let God be truth and all men liars. I was not going to believe the report of a man when God's Word says, "I am the God that healeth thee."

That Sunday, my wife and I went to church with friends of ours. From the beginning of the service, we sensed the presence of the Lord. His presence was strong. During the praise and worship portion of the service, the Pastor did an unusual thing. He stopped the service and said the following, "The Lord told me that all that are sick or have physical need in their bodies should come forward.

As we continued to worship Him, He would heal the sick." That is exactly what happened to me. I felt a heat go through my chest, and I knew that God healed me.

One week later, I returned to the doctor for my follow-up exam. We repeated the process all over again, the X-ray and the blood test. When the results came in, the doctor just shook his head and said, "I see it, but I do not believe it. It is not there anymore."

A great woman of God, Kathryn Kuhlman, saw great. miracles than these take place in her services. The praise and worship lasted as long as two hours before she would get on the platform. When she came on the platform, miracles took place throughout the auditorium. Through her years of ministry, thousands received healing. The most amazing thing is that she rarely laid hands on anyone.

The four ways that God uses to heal mentioned in this chapter are not the only ways that God operates. He can use any way that He sees fit.

"...Not by might, nor by power,

but by my spirit,

saith the Lord of hosts."

Zechariah 4:6 (KJV)

~Chapter 11~
PREVENTATIVE MEDICINE

53

"Do you not discern and understand that you (the whole church) are God's temples [His sanctuary], and that God's Spirit has His permanent dwelling in you [to be at home in you, collectively as a church and also individually]?

If anyone does hurt to God's temple, corrupts it [with false doctrines], or destroys it, God will do hurt to him and bring him to the corruption of death and destroy him. For the temple of God is Holy (sacred to Him) and that [temple} you [the believing church and its individual believers] are." 1 Corinthians 3:16, 17 (AMP)

What must we do to maintain good health in spirit, soul, and body?

- Read God's Word
- Praise without ceasing.
- Pray without ceasing.
- Forsake not the assembling together of the saints.

HEALING SCRIPTURES

FOR THE SPIRIT, SOUL, AND BODY

"Then I lay down and slept in peace and woke up safely, for the Lord was watching over me. And now, although ten thousand enemies surround me on every side, I am not afraid."

Psalm 3:5, 6 (LVB)

"I will lie down in peace and sleep, for though I am alone, O Lord, you will keep me safe."

Psalm 4:8 (LVB)

"The Lord also will be a refuge and a high tower for the oppressed, a refuge and a stronghold in times of trouble (high cost, destitution, and desperation). And they who know Your name [who have experience and acquaintance with Your [mercy] will lean on and confidently put their trust in You, for You, Lord, have not forsaken those who seek (inquire of and for) You [on the authority of God's Word and the right of their necessity].

Psalm 9:9, 10 (AMP)

"O Lord my God, I pleaded with you, and you gave me my health again."

Psalm 30:2 (LVB)

"Oh, how great is Your goodness, which You have laid up
for those who fear, revere, and worship You, goodness which You
have wrought for those who trust and take refuge in You before
the sons of men! In the secret place of Your presence, You hide
them from the plots of men; You keep them secretly in Your
pavilion from the strife of tongues."

Psalm 31:19 – 20 (AMP)

"…For you listened to my plea and answered me. Oh, love
the Lord, all of you who are His people; for the Lord protects those
who are loyal to Him, but harshly punishes all who haughtily
reject Him. So, cheer up! Take courage if you are depending on
the Lord."

Psalm 31:22 -24 (LVB)

"The Angel of the Lord encamps around those who fear
Him [who revere and worship Him with awe] and each of them
He delivers."

Psalm 34:7 (AMP)

"…but those of us who reverence the Lord will never lack
any good thing."

Psalm 34:10 (LVB)

"The good man does not escape all troubles—he has them
too. But the Lord helps him in each and every one.

Psalm 34:19 (LVB)

"Why art thou cast down, O my soul? And why art thou disquieted in me? Hope thou in God: for I shall yet praise Him for the help of His countenance."

Psalm 42:5 (KJV)

"God is our refuge and strength, a very present help in trouble."

Psalm 46:1 (KJV)

"He hath delivered my soul in peace from the battle that was against me: for there were many with me."

Psalm 55:18 (KJV)

"He who dwells in the secret place of the Most High shall remain stable and fixed under the shadow of the Almighty [Whose power no foe can withstand].

Psalm 91:1, 2 (AMP)

"There shall no evil befall you, nor any plague or calamity come near your tent. For He will give His angels [especial] charge over you to accompany and defend and preserve you in all your ways [of obedience and service].

Psalm 91:10, 11 (AMP)

"Who forgives [every one of] all your iniquities, who heals [each one of] all your diseases."

Psalm 103:3 (AMP)

"He shall not be afraid of evil tiding; his heart is firmly fixed, trusting (leaning on and being confident) in the Lord."

Psalm 112:7 (AMP)

"It is vain for you to rise up early, to take rest late, to eat the bread of [anxious] toil – for He gives [blessings] to His beloved in sleep."

Psalm 127:2 (AMP)

"Though I walk amid trouble, You will revive me; You will stretch forth Your hand against the wrath of mine enemies, and Your right hand will save me."

Psalm 138:7 (AMP)

"The Lord opens the eyes of the blind, the Lord lifts those who are bowed down, the Lord loves the [uncompromisingly] righteous (those upright in heart and right standings with Him)."

Psalm 146:8 (AMP)

"Let them praise the name of the Lord: for He commanded, and they were created." (He who created you knows how to heal you.)

Psalm 148:5 (AMP)

"When you lie down, you shall not be afraid; yes, you shall lie down, and your sleep shall be sweet."

Proverbs 3:24 (AMP)

"For the Lord shall be your confidence, firm and strong, and shall keep your foot from being caught [in a trap or some hidden danger].

Proverbs 3:26 (AMP)

"My son, attend to My Words; consent and submit to My sayings. Let them not depart from your sight; keep them in the center of your heart. For they are life to those who find them, healing, and health to all their flesh."

Proverbs 4:20 – 22 (AMP)

"You will guard him and keep him in perfect and constant peace whose mind [both its inclination and its character] is stayed on You because he commits himself to You, leans on You, and hopes confidently in You."

Isaiah 26:3 (AMP)

"…for I will contend with him who contends with you…"

Isaiah 49:25 (AMP)

"Who is among you who [reverently] fears the Lord, who obeys the voice of His Servant, yet who walks in darkness and deep trouble and has no shining splendor [in his heart]? Let him rely on, trust in, and be confident in the name of the Lord, and let him lean upon and be supported by his God."

Isaiah 50:10 (AMP)

"Surely He has borne our griefs (sicknesses, weaknesses and distresses) and carried our sorrows and pains [of punishment] …But He was wounded for our transgressions, He was bruised for our guilt and iniquities; the chastisement (needful to obtain) peace and well-being for us was upon Him; and with the stripes [that wounded] Him we are healed and made whole."

Isaiah 53:4, 5 (AMP)

"You shall establish yourself in righteousness (rightness, in conformity with God's will and order): you shall be far from even the thought of oppression or destruction, for you shall not fear, and from terror, for it shall not come near you."

Isaiah 54:14 (AMP)

"But no weapon that is formed against you shall prosper, and every tongue that shall rise against you in judgment you shall show to be in the wrong…"

Isaiah 54:17 (AMP)

"So shall My word be that goes forth out of My mouth: it shall not return to Me void, [without producing any effect, useless], but it shall accomplish that which I please and purpose, and it shall prosper in the thing for which I sent it." Isaiah 55:11 (AMP)

"…You have seen well, for I am alert and active, watching over My Word to perform it."

Jeremiah 1:12 (AMP)

"For I know the thoughts and plans that I have for you, says the Lord, thoughts, and plans for welfare and peace and not for evil, to give you hope in your outcome. Then you will call upon Me, and you will come and pray to Me, and I will hear and heed you. Then you will seek Me, inquire for, and require Me [as a vital necessity] and find Me when you search for Me with all your heart."

Jeremiah 29:11 – 13 (AMP)

"…He Himself took [in order to carry away] our weaknesses and infirmities and bore away our diseases."

Matthew 8:17 (AMP)

"For verily I say unto you, That whosoever shall say unto this mountain, Be thou removed, and be thou cast into the sea; and shall not doubt in his heart but shall believe that those things which he saith shall come to pass; he shall have whatsoever he saith. Therefore, I say unto you, what things soever ye desire, when ye pray, believe that ye receive them, and ye shall have them."

Mark 11:23, 24 (KJV)

"Give, and [gifts] will be given to you; good measure, pressed down, shaken together, and running over, will t. pour into [the pouch formed by] the bosom [of your robe and used as a bag]. For with the measure, you deal out [with the measure you use when you confer benefits on others], it will be measured back to you.”

Luke 6:38 (AMP)

“Peace I leave with you; My [own] peace I now give to you. Not as the world gives do I give to you. Do not let your hearts be troubled, neither let them be afraid. [Stop allowing yourselves to be agitated and disturbed, and do not permit yourselves to be fearful and intimidated and cowardly and unsettled].”

John 14:27 (AMP)

“He that spared not His own Son, but delivered Him up for us all, how shall He not with Him also freely give us all things?”

Romans 8:32 (KJV)

“Yet amid all these things we are more than conquerors and gain a surpassing victory through Him Who loved us.”

Romans 8:37 (AMP)

“…But we have the mind of Christ (the Messiah) and do hold the thoughts (feelings and purposes) of His heart.”

1 Corinthians 2:16b (AMP)

“Now thanks be unto God, which always causeth us to triumph in Christ, and maketh manifest the savior of His knowledge by us in every place.”

2 Corinthians 2:14 (KJV)

"That He would grant you, according to the riches of His glory, to be strengthened with might by His Spirit in the inner man."

Ephesians 3:16 (KJV)

"And be constantly renewed in the spirit of your mind [having a fresh mental and spiritual attitude]."

Ephesians 4:23 (AMP)

"Wherefore take unto you the whole armor of God, that ye may be able to withstand in the evil day, and having done all, to stand. Stand therefore, having your loins girt about with truth, and having on the breastplate of righteousness; and your feet shod with the preparation of the gospel of peace; above all, taking the shield of faith, wherewith ye shall be able to quench all the fiery darts of the wicked. And take the helmet of salvation, and the sword of the Spirit, which is the word of God: Praying always with all prayer and supplication in the Spirit and watching thereunto with all perseverance and supplication for all saints."

Ephesians 6:13 – 18 (KJV)

"Let this same attitude and purpose and [humble] mind be in you which was in Christ Jesus; [let Him be your example in humility].

Philippians 2: 5 (AMP)

"But my God shall supply all your need according to his riches in glory by Christ Jesus."

Philippians 4:19 (KJV)

"For this cause, we also, since the day we heard it, do not cease to pray for you and to desire that ye might be filled with the knowledge of His will in all wisdom and spiritual understanding. That ye might walk worthy of the Lord unto all pleasing, being fruitful in every good work and increasing in the knowledge of God; Strengthened with all might, according to His glorious power, unto all patience and longsuffering with joyfulness. Giving thanks unto the Father, which hath made us meet to be partakers of the inheritance of the saints in light: Who hath delivered us from the power of darkness, and hath translated us into the kingdom of his dear Son: In whom we have redemption through his blood, even the forgiveness of sins."

Colossians 1:9 – 14 (KJV)

"Yet the Lord is faithful, and He will strengthen [you] and set you on a firm foundation and guard you from the evil [one]."

2 Thessalonians 3:3 (AMP)

"For God did not give us a spirit of timidity (of cowardice, of craven and cringing and fawning fear), but [He has given us a spirit] of power and love and calm and well-balanced mind and discipline and self-control."

2 Timothy 1:7 (AMP)

"Are not the angels all ministering spirits (servants) sent
out in the service [of God for the assistance] of those who are to
inherit salvation?"

Hebrews 1:14 (AMP)

"For the Word that God speaks is alive and full of power
[making it active, operative, energizing, and effective]…We have a
great High Priest Who has [already] ascended and passed through
the heavens, Jesus the Son of God, let us hold fast our confession
[of faith in Him]."

Hebrews 4:12a, 14 (AMP)

"…For He [God] Himself has said, I will not in any way
fail you nor give you up nor leave you without support. [I will] not,
[I will] not, [I will] not in any degree leave you helpless nor
forsake nor let [you] down (relax My hold on you)! [Assuredly
not!] So, we take comfort and are encouraged and confidently and
boldly say, The Lord is my Helper; I will not be seized with alarm
[I will not fear or dread or be terrified]…"

Hebrews 13:5b, 6 (AMP)

"Submit yourselves therefore to God. Resist the devil, and
he will flee from you."

James 4:7 (KJV)

"…by whose stripes ye were healed."

1 Peter 2:24 (KJV)

"…The reason the Son of God was manifest (visible) was to undo (destroy, loosen, and dissolve) the works the devil [has done]."

1 John 3:8 (AMP)

As you read these Scriptures, pray God's Word back to Him. The Anointing that rests upon His Word will go forth and accomplish God's results, His purpose, and plans, because the Anointing has destroyed the yoke.

HINDRANCES TO PRAYER

1. "Examine yourselves, whether ye be in the faith; prove yourselves."   2 Corinthians 13:5a; (1 Cor. 11:31)

2. "If we confess our sins, He is faithful and just to forgive us our sins and to cleanse us from all unrighteousness."   1 John 1:9 (Matt. 16:19; Matt. 18:18; 1 Sam. 15:22; Matt. 5:23–24; Matt. 18:21-22; Mk. 11:25-26; Luke 23:34; Jn. 20:23; 2 Cor. 2:10-11; Ps. 32:1-5)

3. "If ye be willing and obedient, ye shall eat the good of the land." Isaiah 1:19 (Mk. 12:30-31; Matt. 22:36-40; Jas. 4:17; Josh. 7; Deut. 7:25-26; Deut. 5:16)

4. "There is therefore now no condemnation to them which are in Christ Jesus, who walk not after the flesh, but after the Spirit." Romans 8:1 (Jn. 3:17; Phil. 1:6; 1 Pet. 5:7; Prov. 26:24-28; 1 Jn. 2:9-12; 1 Jn. 3:15-22)

5. "And Jesus said unto the centurion: Go thy way; and as thou hast believed, so be it done unto thee. And his servant was healed in the selfsame hour." Matthew 8:13 (Jas. 5:15; Mk. 16:16-18; Jn. 7:37-39; Prov. 3:5-7; Heb. 4:6; Heb. 3:12; Rom. 4:20-21; Isa. 7:9)

6. **Pray Correctly**: "Be careful about nothing, but in everything by prayer and supplication with thanksgiving let your requests be made known unto God." Philippians 4:6 (1 Thess. 5:18; Eph. 5:20-21; Ps. 100:4)

   "I exhort therefore, that, first of all, supplications, prayers, intercessions, and giving of thanks, be made for all men; For kings, and for all that are in authority; that we may lead a quiet and peaceable life in all godliness and honesty. For this is good and acceptable in the sight of God our Savior, Who will have all men to be saved, and to come unto the knowledge of the truth. 1 Timothy 2:1 – 4

"…for I watch over my Word to perform it." Jeremiah 1:12 (ASV) Isa. 55:11; Hos. 14:2

7. "He that turneth away his ear from hearing the law, even his prayer shall be abomination." Proverbs 28:9

8. "If ye abide in me, and my words abide in you, ye shall ask what ye will, and it shall be done unto you." John 15:7 (Job 22:28)

9. "But take heed to yourselves, lest your souls be weighed down with self-indulgence and drunkenness or the anxieties of this life, and that day come upon you, suddenly, like a falling trap…" Luke 21:34 (Weymouth's NT) (1 Cor. 9:25-27; Rom. 12:1-2; Prov. 23:1-3; 6-8)

10. "Saying, Touch not mine anointed, and do my prophets no harm." Psalms 105:15 (1 Chr. 16:22; 1 Sam. 26:5-11; 1 Thess. 5:12-13; Heb. 6:10)

11. "In God will I praise His Word; in God, I put my confidence: I will not fear; what can flesh do unto me?" Psalms 56:4 (Darby's Bible)(Isa. 51:7, 12; Job 22:28; Ps. 111:10; Prov. 29:25; Prov. 2:1-5; Ps. 56:4, 11; Mal. 3:16-18; 4:2; Isa. 29:13-14; 2 Tim. 1:7; 1 Jn. 4:18; Rev. 12:11)

12. "Will a man rob God? Yet ye have robbed me. But ye say, Wherein have we robbed thee? In tithes and offerings. Ye are cursed with a curse: for ye have robbed me, even this whole nation. Bring ye all the tithes into the storehouse, that there may be meat in mine house, and prove me now herewith, saith the Lord of hosts, if I will not open you the windows of heaven, and pour you out a blessing, that there shall not be room enough to receive it." Malachi 3:8-10 (Lev. 27:30-32; Josh. 7; Josh. 6:19; 2 Cor. 9:6-10; Prov. 3:9-10; Lk. 6:38; Rom. 12:13; 1 Cor. 9:13; Num. 8:24-32)

13. "Wherefore whosoever shall eat this bread, and drink this cup of the Lord, unworthily, shall be guilty of the body and blood of the Lord. But let a man examine himself, and so let him eat of that bread, and drink of that cup. For he, that hateth and drinketh unworthily, hateth and drinketh damnation to himself, not

discerning the Lord's body. For this cause, many are weak and sickly among you, and many sleep. For if we would judge ourselves, we should not be judged." 1 Corinthians 11:27-31 (Eph. 4:29-32; Jas. 4:11; Rom. 15:1-7; Gal. 5:26; Heb. 10:24)

14. "So, then faith cometh by hearing, and hearing by the Word of God." Rom. 10:17 (Matt. 9:27-29; Mk. 5:25-34; Lk. 1:45; Rom. 4:21; Heb. 10:23; Lk 22:42; Mk. 14:36)

15. "The good men perish; the godly die before their time and no one seems to care or wonder why. No one seems to realize that God is taking them away from evil days ahead." Isaiah 57:1 (LVB)

16. "To everything there is a season, and a time to every purpose under the heaven: A time to be born, and a time to die; a time to plant, and a time to pluck up that which is planted." Eccl. 3:1-2) (Heb. 9:27; Isa. 55:8-9)

ABOUT FRANK BAIO

Frank Baio is an anointed and gifted man of God. He is sensitive to the Holy Spirit and flows with the Spirit. In every service, the Holy Spirit manifests Himself powerfully. God confirms His Word with miracles, signs, and wonders.

God showed Frank that the Church of Jesus Christ is hurting. Frank has been called to help bring about healing by helping the church to:

- Experience the different levels of worship.
- reach its maximum potential in ministry.
- Develop a deeper prayer life.
- Learn Spiritual Warfare

In October of 1988, the Lord spoke to Frank's heart for 24 hours. He could not eat, sleep, or drink because of the intense anointing over him. This is what the Lord said:

"Arise, my son, for now, is the time for which I have been preparing you. I, the Lord your God, am with you. I will never leave you nor forsake you. I have called you to preach and teach My Word to My people. I, the Lord, will change the lives of those who hear and obey My Word. I will cause them to be victorious. I will bring about healing in their hearts and lives and wherever they go. My son, my call has been upon you from childhood. Now, choose you this day whom you will serve."

- Frank and his wife, Fran, have been married for since 1969.
- Frank has pastored churches for 7 years.
- Bible Institute Teacher at Christian Retreat, Bradenton, FL
- Praise and Worship seminars.
- Church Leadership Seminars
- Marriage Seminars

- Missions Trip to Haiti – 75 Churches Established

- Missions Trip to Jamaica

- Taught Pastors in Haiti at the School of Ministry

- Conference Speaker

Frank and Fran are available for Ministry.

CONTACT INFORMATION:

Frank Baio Ministries

921 Faith Circle East, #70

Bradenton, Florida 34212

Phone/FAX # 941-779-8324.

E-mail baioministries@verizon.net

www.baioministries.com